CLINICAL INSIGHTS IN SPORTS MEDICINE

From Diagnosis to Ethical Decisions

Dr Essam Abdelhakim

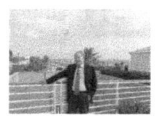

CONTENTS

INTRODUCTION

Sports Medicine is a dynamic and evolving field that bridges the gap between medicine, surgery, and rehabilitation, focusing on the prevention, diagnosis, and management of injuries related to physical activity and exercise.

With the increasing emphasis on fitness, competitive sports, and active lifestyles, the role of sports medicine has expanded far beyond treating athletes it now includes individuals of all ages and activity levels.

*This book provides a **comprehensive yet concise review of essential topics in sports medicine**, ranging from musculoskeletal injuries, joint disorders, and overuse syndromes to exercise physiology, sports nutrition, and injury prevention strategies. Each topic is structured to highlight **key definitions, clinical presentation, diagnostic approaches, management options, and prognosis**, ensuring clarity and exam relevance.*

Designed for **medical students, residents, and healthcare professionals**, this resource is equally valuable for those preparing for **licensing and specialty exams** as well as clinicians seeking practical guidance in the care of active patients.

1. INTRODUCTION TO SPORTS MEDICINE

Overview and History of Sports Medicine

Sports Medicine is a rapidly growing discipline focused on physical fitness, the treatment and prevention of sports-related injuries, and overall health promotion for athletes and active individuals.

Historically, sports medicine evolved in response to the need for specialized care to manage injuries resulting from physical activity and competitive sports.

Its origins can be traced back to ancient civilizations; for instance, physicians in ancient Greece, like Galen, treated gladiators and emphasized the importance of exercise in promoting health.

The modern foundation of sports medicine was laid in the 20th century, driven by advances in understanding human anatomy, physiology, and the mechanics of physical performance.

Notably, major sports events like the Olympic Games and the growing popularity of professional sports highlighted the need for specialized healthcare providers focused on optimizing athletes' performance and recovery.

By the mid-20th century, sports medicine had expanded to encompass the prevention, diagnosis, treatment, and rehabilitation of sports injuries, ultimately forming a unique and multifaceted medical field.

Today, sports medicine is recognized as a critical component of healthcare, benefiting not only elite athletes but also recreational athletes, individuals pursuing fitness, and people recovering from physical injuries.

The specialty emphasizes evidence-based care and collaboration between healthcare providers, aiming to maximize physical function and improve patients' quality of life.

Role Of The Sports Medicine Physician

Their responsibilities encompass:

1. **Injury Diagnosis and Treatment**: Sports medicine physicians have extensive training in diagnosing sports-related injuries, such as ligament sprains, muscle strains, fractures, and concussions. Treatment options often include conservative management like physical therapy, bracing, medications, and minimally invasive interventions.

2. **Injury Prevention**: Preventing injury is a major focus. Physicians design and implement personalized conditioning programs, teach proper exercise techniques, and collaborate with athletic trainers and coaches to minimize injury risks.

3. **Rehabilitation and Return-to-Play**: These professionals oversee an athlete's rehabilitation, ensuring a safe and effective return to their activity level. They work with physical therapists to tailor programs that restore strength, mobility, and endurance.

4. **Optimizing Athletic Performance**: Beyond injury care, sports medicine physicians offer expertise in nutrition, exercise physiology, mental health support, and performance optimization strategies tailored to each individual's goals.

5. **Education and Advocacy**: Educating athletes, coaches, and the general public about safe exercise practices and proper recovery methods is another key area. They also advocate for safer sports environments and the ethical use of performance-enhancing treatments.

Multidisciplinary Approach To Sports Medicine Care

This approach typically involves:

1. **Orthopedic Surgeons**: In cases where surgical intervention is necessary (e.g., ligament reconstructions or fracture repairs), orthopedic surgeons bring their expertise to restore structural integrity and function.

2. **Physical Therapists**: They design and implement rehabilitation protocols, focusing on regaining strength, flexibility, balance, and functional capacity.

3. **Athletic Trainers**: As frontline responders, they often assess injuries during athletic events, provide initial care, and assist with rehabilitation and injury prevention.

4. **Nutritionists/Dietitians**: Proper nutrition is crucial for performance and recovery. Nutritionists provide tailored dietary recommendations for athletes, addressing needs for energy, recovery, weight management, and specific goals like muscle building or endurance.

5. **Sports Psychologists**: The mental aspect of sports can significantly impact an athlete's performance. Sports psychologists help athletes cope with stress, enhance focus, build confidence, and recover from the psychological toll of injuries.

6. **Primary Care Physicians and Specialists**: Cardiology, endocrinology, and other specialties may be involved when athletes present with medical conditions that intersect with their physical activity.

ESSAM ABDELHAKIM

2. ANATOMY AND BIOMECHANICS OF MOVEMENT IN SPORTS

Basic Musculoskeletal Anatomy Relevant To Sports

Key components include:

1. **Bones**: The skeletal system provides structural support, acts as a lever system for muscles, and protects vital organs. Long bones like the femur, humerus, and tibia are particularly important in weight-bearing and movement. Sports activities often stress bones, potentially leading to stress fractures or other injuries.

2. **Muscles**: Skeletal muscles generate force and motion. They are classified into different types based on their role, such as:

   - **Prime Movers (Agonists)**: Responsible for initiating movement, such as the quadriceps during leg extension.
   - **Antagonists**: Muscles that oppose the action of the agonist, such as the hamstrings during knee extension.
   - **Synergists**: Assist the prime movers by adding extra force or stabilizing the movement.
   - **Stabilizers**: Contract to maintain posture and control during movement, like the core muscles during a squat.

3. **Tendons and Ligaments**:
    - **Tendons** connect muscle to bone, transmitting the force generated by muscle contraction to create movement. Tendon injuries, such as tendinopathies, are common in sports due to repetitive loading.
    - **Ligaments** connect bone to bone and stabilize joints, preventing excessive motion. Ligament injuries (e.g., ACL tears) often occur due to sudden changes in direction, stops, or contact.
4. **Joints**: Joints are points where bones meet and allow for different ranges of motion, classified based on their structure and mobility (e.g., hinge joints, ball-and-socket joints). Joint stability and mobility are critical in sports performance, and imbalances can lead to injury.
5. **Cartilage**: Articular cartilage covers the ends of bones within joints, reducing friction and absorbing shock. Cartilage injuries, such as meniscal tears or osteochondral lesions, can significantly impact an athlete's performance.

Kinematics And Kinetics Of Human Movement

To understand movement mechanics in sports, we must explore **kinematics** *(the study of motion without regard to forces) and* **kinetics** *(the study of forces that cause or change motion).*

1. **Kinematics**:
    - **Linear and Angular Motion**: Sports movements can involve linear (straight-line) motion, such as sprinting, or angular motion, such as a gymnast rotating around a bar.
    - **Velocity and Acceleration**: The speed

and direction of an athlete's movements influence performance. For example, increasing sprint velocity requires optimal muscle activation, stride length, and frequency.

- **Displacement**: This refers to the change in position of an athlete's body segments during motion and is crucial in sports such as swimming and cycling.

2. **Kinetics**:

- **Force**: This is a push or pull exerted on an object or body. Muscular force, ground reaction force (GRF), and impact forces (e.g., landing from a jump) significantly influence performance and injury risk.

- **Torque**: The rotational equivalent of force; it determines how effectively an athlete can rotate around a joint axis. Understanding torque is essential in movements like throwing, kicking, or pivoting.

- **Impulse**: The product of force and the time it is applied; it plays a role in activities like weightlifting and sprint starts, where maximizing force over a short period is beneficial.

Understanding Biomechanical Load And Sports Performance

Biomechanical load refers to the forces exerted on tissues, bones, and joints during physical activity.

Proper load management is crucial for optimizing performance and preventing injuries.

Key considerations include:

1. **Loading Patterns**: Different sports impose unique loading demands. Runners experience repeated impact loads on the lower extremities, while baseball pitchers encounter high rotational and tensile loads on the shoulder and elbow joints. Understanding these patterns allows practitioners to create tailored training and injury prevention plans.

2. **Overload and Adaptation**: The concept of progressive overload—gradually increasing stress on the body—stimulates adaptation and performance improvements. However, excessive load without adequate recovery can lead to overuse injuries, such as tendinopathies and stress fractures.

3. **Muscle Balance and Alignment**: Imbalances in muscle strength and joint alignment can lead to inefficient movement patterns and higher injury risk. For instance, weak gluteal muscles may lead to knee valgus during squats and increase ACL injury risk.

4. **Ground Reaction Forces (GRFs)**: In sports such as running and jumping, GRFs play a critical role in performance and injury. Proper landing mechanics can reduce impact forces and injury risk, highlighting the importance of training proper techniques.

5. **Load Distribution and Fatigue**: Proper distribution of load across joints and tissues minimizes localized stress. Fatigue alters biomechanical movement patterns, potentially increasing injury risk, emphasizing the need for conditioning programs.

6. **Performance Optimization**: Understanding biomechanics allows for fine-tuning of techniques to maximize athletic output. Examples include perfecting a golfer's swing to increase clubhead speed while minimizing back strain or optimizing running gait for speed and efficiency.

3. GENERAL PRINCIPLES OF SPORTS INJURIES

Classification Of Sports Injuries: Acute Vs. Chronic

Sports injuries *are commonly classified into two major categories: acute and chronic, based on their onset, duration, and underlying mechanisms.*

1. **Acute Injuries:**
   - **Definition**: Acute injuries occur suddenly due to a specific event or trauma, often during physical activity. They typically involve a recognizable mechanism of injury, such as a collision, fall, or twisting movement.
   - **Common Examples**:
     - **Sprains**: Ligament injuries, such as an ankle sprain, typically caused by excessive stretching or tearing.
     - **Strains**: Muscle or tendon injuries, like a hamstring strain, resulting from overstretching or sudden forceful contractions.
     - **Fractures**: Breaks in bones caused by sudden impact or high force, such as during a fall.
     - **Dislocations**: The displacement of a bone from its normal joint position, often seen in shoulder or finger injuries.

- **Contusions (Bruises)**: Result from a direct impact that damages the soft tissues and causes localized bleeding.

2. **Chronic Injuries**:

   ○ **Definition**: Chronic injuries, often referred to as "overuse injuries," develop gradually over time due to repeated stress or prolonged activity. These injuries often result from biomechanical imbalances, poor training techniques, or inadequate recovery.

   ○ **Common Examples**:

      - **Tendinopathies**: Chronic tendon injuries such as Achilles tendinopathy or tennis elbow, characterized by pain, swelling, and stiffness.

      - **Stress Fractures**: Tiny cracks in bones caused by repetitive stress, common in weight-bearing activities like running.

      - **Shin Splints (Medial Tibial Stress Syndrome)**: Pain and inflammation along the inner border of the shinbone due to repeated impact or stress.

      - **Plantar Fasciitis**: Chronic inflammation of the plantar fascia, causing heel pain, often due to prolonged standing or excessive running.

Mechanisms Of Sports Injuries

Some common mechanisms include:

1. **Direct Trauma**:
   - Injuries resulting from direct impact or contact, such as being struck by an object (e.g., a ball or opponent). Examples include contusions, fractures, and dislocations.

2. **Indirect Trauma**:
   - Caused by forces transmitted through the body, often without direct contact. Examples include ACL tears from sudden deceleration or pivoting movements.

3. **Overstretching or Overloading**:
   - Excessive stretching of muscles, tendons, or ligaments beyond their normal range can result in sprains or strains. This often occurs during explosive or rapid movements.

4. **Repetitive Stress**:
   - Repeated low-grade stress over time leads to chronic injuries. Poor technique, inappropriate equipment, or training errors can exacerbate these stresses. For instance, repetitive overhead motions can cause rotator cuff injuries in swimmers and pitchers.

5. **Poor Biomechanics**:
   - Faulty movement patterns, such as improper running gait or poor posture, place excessive strain on certain structures and increase the risk of injury.

6. **Environmental Factors**:
   - Surfaces (e.g., hard vs. soft ground), footwear, and weather conditions can contribute to injury risk. Slippery or uneven

surfaces may lead to slips and falls.

The Role Of Overuse And Repetitive Stress

Overuse injuries *result from the accumulation of repetitive stress on tissues without adequate time for recovery and repair.*

These injuries are prevalent in sports that involve continuous, high-frequency movements, such as running, cycling, swimming, or tennis.

Key contributors to overuse injuries include:

1. **Training Errors**:
   - Sudden increases in training volume, intensity, or duration without gradual adaptation.
   - Insufficient rest periods or recovery time between workouts.

2. **Poor Technique**:
   - Faulty movement patterns, like improper running mechanics, can place excess stress on joints and muscles.

3. **Muscle Imbalances**:
   - Weakness or tightness in certain muscle groups alters biomechanics and increases the risk of injury. For example, weak hip stabilizers may contribute to knee pain in runners.

4. **Inadequate Equipment**:
   - Worn-out or inappropriate footwear, for example, can lead to foot, ankle, and lower leg injuries.

5. **Intrinsic Factors**:
   - Factors such as age, previous injuries, and individual anatomy (e.g., flat feet or hypermobility) can influence the risk of

developing chronic injuries.

Managing overuse injuries *requires a multifaceted approach that addresses both the underlying cause and the symptoms.*

Interventions may include rest, activity modification, physical therapy, strength training, and biomechanical analysis.

Injury Prevention Strategies And Programs

Effective injury prevention programs consider the specific demands of each sport and individual athlete needs.

1. **Proper Warm-Up and Cool-Down**:
   - A structured warm-up increases blood flow, raises muscle temperature, and prepares the body for activity, reducing the risk of acute injuries. Cool-down exercises, including stretching, promote recovery.

2. **Strength and Conditioning**:
   - Building muscle strength and endurance improves joint stability, reduces fatigue, and prevents injuries. Specific strength training programs target sport-specific movements and reduce biomechanical stress.

3. **Flexibility and Mobility Training**:
   - Stretching exercises and mobility drills maintain or improve range of motion, reducing stiffness and preventing muscle strains.

4. **Correct Technique and Biomechanical Training**:
   - Athletes benefit from proper coaching to ensure correct technique during sports movements. Addressing faulty biomechanics can reduce stress on joints and soft tissues.

5. **Adequate Rest and Recovery**:
   - Rest days and recovery periods between training sessions allow tissues to repair and adapt, reducing the risk of chronic injuries.

6. **Progressive Overload**:
   - Gradually increasing the intensity, volume, and frequency of training allows for physiological adaptations without overstressing tissues.

7. **Use of Protective Equipment**:
   - Helmets, padding, braces, and other protective gear minimize the risk of direct trauma injuries.

8. **Balanced Training Programs**:
   - Cross-training and alternating types of physical activities can reduce repetitive stress on specific structures and prevent overuse injuries.

9. **Monitoring Workload**:
   - Tracking training loads, fatigue levels, and overall well-being helps identify early signs of overtraining and mitigate injury risk.

10. **Education and Awareness**:
   - Athletes, coaches, and healthcare professionals should be educated about injury risks, signs of overtraining, and prevention strategies.

4. DIAGNOSTIC TOOLS AND TECHNIQUES IN SPORTS MEDICINE

Clinical History And Examination

Key elements of this process include:

1. **Patient History**:
    - **Chief Complaint**: Detailed description of symptoms (pain, swelling, instability, etc.), onset, duration, and character.
    - **Mechanism of Injury**: Understanding how the injury occurred (e.g., trauma, sudden twist, repetitive stress).
    - **History of Previous Injuries**: Past injuries can influence the current condition and reveal predisposing factors.
    - **Training and Activity Level**: Information about training regimen, frequency, intensity, type of sport, and workload.
    - **Medical History**: Pre-existing medical conditions, medications, and relevant surgical history.
    - **Psychosocial Context**: Consideration of mental health, stressors, and motivation, which can impact recovery and performance.
2. **Physical Examination**:

- **Inspection**: Visual assessment for swelling, discoloration, deformities, muscle atrophy, and scars.
- **Palpation**: Assessing tenderness, warmth, swelling, crepitus, or deformity by physically examining the affected region.
- **Range of Motion (ROM)**: Evaluating both active and passive movement to identify limitations or abnormalities.
- **Strength Testing**: Measuring muscle strength through resisted movements.
- **Stability Tests**: Assessing joint stability using specific maneuvers (e.g., Lachman test for ACL integrity).
- **Special Tests**: Sport-specific maneuvers to evaluate specific structures (e.g., McMurray's test for meniscal injuries).
- **Neurological Assessment**: Testing for sensory, motor, and reflex deficits.

Imaging Modalities: X-Rays, Mri, Ultrasound, And Ct Scans

Common imaging modalities include:

1. **X-rays**:
    - **Description**: Standard radiographs use low-dose ionizing radiation to capture images of bones.
    - **Uses**: Ideal for detecting fractures, dislocations, bone alignment, and joint space narrowing (e.g., arthritis).
    - **Limitations**: Limited soft tissue visualization and may miss stress fractures

or early-stage bone injuries.

2. **Magnetic Resonance Imaging (MRI)**:

   - **Description**: MRI uses powerful magnets and radio waves to generate detailed images of soft tissues, bones, and organs.
   - **Uses**: Highly sensitive for diagnosing ligament tears (e.g., ACL), muscle injuries, cartilage damage, tendinopathies, and joint pathology.
   - **Advantages**: Non-invasive with excellent soft tissue contrast, making it suitable for complex or ambiguous injuries.
   - **Limitations**: Costly, not always available, and contraindicated for some patients (e.g., those with certain implants).

3. **Ultrasound (US)**:

   - **Description**: Real-time imaging technique that uses high-frequency sound waves to visualize muscles, tendons, and other soft tissues.
   - **Uses**: Portable and cost-effective, used to diagnose tendon injuries, muscle tears, bursitis, and to guide injections or therapeutic interventions.
   - **Advantages**: Allows dynamic assessments (e.g., observing muscle contractions) and provides immediate results.
   - **Limitations**: Operator-dependent with limited depth penetration; less effective for visualizing deep or complex structures.

4. **Computed Tomography (CT) Scans**:

   - **Description**: CT uses rotating X-ray beams and computer processing to produce cross-sectional images of bones, organs, and other structures.

- **Uses**: Detailed imaging of complex bone fractures, joint surfaces, and in cases where precise anatomical definition is required.
- **Advantages**: Fast imaging, making it useful in acute trauma settings.
- **Limitations**: Higher radiation exposure compared to X-rays, limited soft tissue contrast relative to MRI.

Functional Testing And Biomechanical Assessments

Functional and biomechanical assessments analyze an athlete's movement patterns, strength, flexibility, and coordination to understand injury mechanisms and guide rehabilitation.

1. **Functional Movement Screening (FMS):**
   - Assesses fundamental movement patterns to identify mobility and stability deficits.
   - Useful for identifying athletes at risk for injuries and creating individualized training plans.

2. **Gait Analysis:**
   - Involves detailed assessment of walking or running mechanics, often using video or motion capture systems.
   - Commonly used to identify issues in runners or evaluate lower limb injuries.

3. **Balance and Proprioception Testing:**
   - Assesses an athlete's ability to maintain stability and react to perturbations, crucial in sports that demand agility and

coordination.

4. **Strength Testing with Dynamometry**:
   - Quantifies muscle strength to evaluate deficits and monitor rehabilitation progress.

5. **Force Plate Analysis**:
   - Measures ground reaction forces during activities like jumping or landing, providing insights into load distribution and symmetry.

Laboratory Tests And Biomarkers In Sports Injuries

Laboratory tests are sometimes necessary to assess metabolic, inflammatory, or immune-related conditions that affect athletes.

1. **Markers of Muscle Damage**:
   - **Creatine Kinase (CK)** and **Lactate Dehydrogenase (LDH)**: Elevated levels indicate muscle breakdown or overtraining.

2. **Inflammatory Markers**:
   - **C-Reactive Protein (CRP)** and **Erythrocyte Sedimentation Rate (ESR)**: Elevated levels suggest inflammation, infection, or chronic overuse.

3. **Hormonal and Metabolic Profiles**:
   - Assessment of **hormones** (e.g., cortisol, testosterone) can help evaluate fatigue, overtraining syndrome, or nutritional deficiencies.

4. **Bone Health Assessments**:

- Tests like **Vitamin D levels**, **calcium**, and **bone mineral density (BMD)** tests, such as **DEXA scans**, are relevant in stress fractures and conditions affecting bone metabolism.

5. **Genetic Testing** (emerging field):

- Identifies genetic markers linked to performance, injury susceptibility, or recovery rates, guiding individualized training.

5. MANAGEMENT OF COMMON SPORTS INJURIES

Treatment strategies depend on the type and severity of the injury and involve multidisciplinary care tailored to the specific needs of each patient.

a. Soft Tissue Injuries

1. **Sprains, Strains, and Contusions:**

   - **Sprains** involve ligament injuries, often resulting from stretching or tearing due to joint overload or twisting forces (e.g., ankle sprains).

   - **Strains** are injuries to muscles or tendons caused by overstretching or excessive force (e.g., hamstring strain).

   - **Contusions (bruises)** occur due to direct trauma, leading to localized bleeding and swelling.

   - **Management:**

     - **RICE Protocol** (Rest, Ice, Compression, Elevation): Initial treatment for reducing pain and inflammation.

     - **Immobilization:** Splinting or bracing for moderate to severe injuries.

     - **Rehabilitation:** Gradual progression through physical therapy to restore strength, range of motion (ROM), and function.

2. **Tendinopathies (Tennis Elbow, Achilles Tendinopathy, etc.):**
   - **Description**: Chronic tendon conditions due to overuse, characterized by pain, stiffness, and swelling.
   - **Management**:
     - **Activity Modification**: Reducing activities that worsen symptoms.
     - **Eccentric Strengthening**: Exercises specifically targeting tendon rehabilitation.
     - **Physical Therapy**: Modalities like ultrasound therapy or shockwave therapy.
     - **Medications**: NSAIDs (Non-Steroidal Anti-Inflammatory Drugs) for symptom relief.
     - **Advanced Therapies**: Corticosteroid injections or platelet-rich plasma (PRP) therapy may be considered.

3. **Ligament Tears (ACL, MCL, LCL):**
   - **Anterior Cruciate Ligament (ACL)** injuries are common in athletes involved in pivoting sports.
   - **Medial and Lateral Collateral Ligament (MCL, LCL)** injuries may result from direct impact or stress to the knee joint.
   - **Management**:
     - **Partial Tears**: Conservative care with bracing, physical therapy, and strengthening.
     - **Complete Tears**: Often require

surgical repair or reconstruction (e.g., ACL reconstruction).

- **Rehabilitation**: Comprehensive program to regain stability, mobility, and neuromuscular control.

4. **Bursitis**:

   ◦ **Description**: Inflammation of the bursa, often due to repetitive movement or prolonged pressure.

   ◦ **Common Sites**: Shoulder (subacromial bursitis), knee (prepatellar bursitis), and elbow (olecranon bursitis).

   ◦ **Management**:

     - **Rest and Ice**: Reduces acute inflammation.
     - **NSAIDs**: Alleviate pain and swelling.
     - **Physical Therapy**: Stretching, strengthening, and modifying activities.
     - **Aspiration or Injection**: In cases of significant swelling or non-responsiveness to conservative measures.

b. Bone and Joint Injuries

1. **Fractures (Stress Fractures, Avulsion Fractures, etc.)**:

   ◦ **Stress Fractures**: Result from repetitive microtrauma, common in endurance athletes (e.g., tibia, metatarsals).

   ◦ **Avulsion Fractures**: Occur when a tendon or ligament pulls off a piece of bone, often in high-impact activities.

- ○ **Management**:
  - **Immobilization**: Casting or bracing to facilitate healing.
  - **Activity Modification**: Cessation of high-impact activities.
  - **Surgical Fixation**: Indicated for unstable or complex fractures.
  - **Bone Health Optimization**: Addressing nutrition, calcium, and vitamin D levels.

2. **Dislocations and Subluxations**:
   - ○ **Description**: Joint displacement (complete or partial), often due to high-energy trauma.
   - ○ **Common Sites**: Shoulder, patella, fingers, and hip.
   - ○ **Management**:
     - **Reduction**: Manual repositioning of the joint.
     - **Immobilization**: Bracing to prevent recurrence.
     - **Rehabilitation**: Strengthening surrounding muscles to maintain joint stability.
     - **Surgical Intervention**: Necessary for recurrent or complex dislocations.

3. **Cartilage Injuries (Meniscal Tears, Osteochondral Lesions)**:
   - ○ **Meniscal Tears**: Common in twisting injuries of the knee.
   - ○ **Osteochondral Lesions**: Damage to the

cartilage and underlying bone due to trauma.

- ○ **Management**:
    - ▪ **Conservative**: Rest, NSAIDs, and physical therapy.
    - ▪ **Surgical Options**: Arthroscopic repair, meniscectomy, or cartilage restoration procedures.
    - ▪ **Rehabilitation**: Focused on ROM, strength, and stability restoration.

c. Muscle Injuries

1. **Muscle Tears (Hamstring, Calf, Quadriceps)**:
    - ○ **Grades**: Vary from minor strains (Grade I) to complete ruptures (Grade III).
    - ○ **Management**:
        - ▪ **Acute Phase**: RICE, NSAIDs, and protective bracing.
        - ▪ **Rehabilitation**: Progressive strengthening, stretching, and return-to-play criteria.

2. **Compartment Syndrome**:
    - ○ **Description**: Increased pressure within a muscle compartment, reducing blood flow and potentially leading to ischemia.
    - ○ **Management**:
        - ▪ **Acute Compartment Syndrome**: Requires **emergency fasciotomy**.
        - ▪ **Chronic Exertional Compartment Syndrome**: Conservative management with activity modification or surgical release.

3. **Muscle Cramps and Myositis**:

- **Management of Cramps**: Hydration, electrolyte balance, stretching, and addressing underlying triggers.
- **Myositis (Inflammatory Muscle Conditions)**: May require **immune-modulating therapies** and rehabilitation.

d. Specific Joint Injuries

1. Shoulder:

- **Rotator Cuff Tear**: Often results from repetitive overhead activities.
  - **Management**: Rest, physiotherapy, corticosteroid injections, or surgical repair.
- **Shoulder Dislocation**: High risk of recurrence in athletes.
  - **Management**: Reduction, immobilization, and rehabilitation; surgery for recurrent cases.
- **Labral Tear (SLAP Lesions)**:
  - **Management**: Conservative care or surgical repair depending on severity.

2. Knee:

- **Meniscal Injuries**: Twisting forces often cause damage.
  - **Management**: Conservative or surgical depending on the tear's location and severity.
- **Patellofemoral Pain Syndrome (Runner's Knee)**:
  - **Management**: Strengthening, orthotics, and activity modification.

3. **Ankle and Foot**:

- **Ankle Sprains**: Common in sports, often involving lateral ligament injury.
  - **Management**: RICE, bracing, and rehabilitation.
- **Plantar Fasciitis**: Chronic heel pain due to plantar fascia strain.
  - **Management**: Stretching, orthotics, and activity modification.
- **Achilles Tendon Rupture**:
  - **Management**: Conservative casting or surgical repair.

4. **Elbow and Hand**:

- **Golfer's Elbow (Medial Epicondylitis)**:
  - **Management**: Rest, strengthening exercises, and bracing.
- **Carpal Tunnel Syndrome**:
  - **Management**: Splinting, activity modification, or surgical release.
- **Wrist Sprain**:
  - **Management**: Immobilization, physical therapy, and rehabilitation.

6. SPECIAL CONSIDERATIONS IN SPORTS INJURIES

Concussions And Sports-Related Head Injuries

1. **Overview**:
   - Concussions are a form of mild traumatic brain injury (TBI) caused by direct or indirect impact to the head, resulting in transient neurological impairment.
   - Common in contact sports such as football, rugby, hockey, and boxing.

2. **Symptoms**:
   - Physical: Headache, dizziness, nausea, balance disturbances.
   - Cognitive: Confusion, memory loss, difficulty concentrating.
   - Emotional: Mood changes, irritability, anxiety.
   - Sleep: Sleep disturbances or drowsiness.

3. **Diagnosis**:
   - Clinical evaluation using standardized tools such as the **SCAT5 (Sports Concussion Assessment Tool)**.
   - Neurological examination and cognitive assessment.
   - Imaging (CT, MRI) may be used in cases

of suspected structural injury or prolonged symptoms.

4. **Management**:

- ◦ **Immediate Removal**: Athletes suspected of having a concussion should be removed from play immediately.
- ◦ **Rest and Gradual Return to Activity**: Physical and cognitive rest is recommended, followed by a stepwise return-to-play protocol.
- ◦ **Monitoring and Follow-Up**: Close observation for persistent symptoms and potential post-concussion syndrome.
- ◦ **Prevention**: Use of protective gear, education on safe play, and adherence to sports-specific concussion protocols.

Heat-Related Illnesses And Dehydration

1. **Heat Illnesses in Sports**:

- ◦ **Heat Cramps**: Painful muscle spasms due to loss of electrolytes and dehydration.
- ◦ **Heat Exhaustion**: Characterized by excessive sweating, weakness, nausea, and dizziness due to prolonged heat exposure.
- ◦ **Heat Stroke**: A life-threatening condition with high body temperature, confusion, altered mental status, and possible organ damage.

2. **Risk Factors**:

- ◦ High ambient temperatures, high humidity, poor hydration, lack of acclimatization, and intense physical activity.

3. **Management**:
  - **Heat Cramps**: Rest, hydration with electrolyte-rich fluids, stretching, and cooling.
  - **Heat Exhaustion**: Move the athlete to a cooler environment, apply cooling measures, and hydrate orally or intravenously.
  - **Heat Stroke: Medical emergency requiring immediate action**—rapid cooling (e.g., ice packs, immersion in cold water), IV fluids, and emergency transport.
  - **Prevention**: Adequate hydration strategies, gradual acclimatization, and heat index monitoring during training and competition.

4. **Dehydration**:
  - **Symptoms**: Thirst, dry mouth, decreased urine output, weakness, and impaired performance.
  - **Prevention and Management**: Monitoring hydration status, electrolyte replacement, and personalized hydration plans based on individual sweat rates.

Cold Weather And Altitude-Related Conditions

1. **Cold-Related Injuries**:
  - **Frostbite**: Freezing of skin and underlying tissues, commonly affecting fingers, toes, ears, and nose.
    - **Management**: Gradual rewarming, protecting the affected area, and

medical evaluation.

- **Hypothermia**: Lowered core body temperature due to prolonged cold exposure.
  - **Management**: Immediate warming, dry clothing, and hospital care if severe.

2. **Altitude-Related Conditions**:
   - **Acute Mountain Sickness (AMS)**: Symptoms include headache, nausea, and fatigue due to rapid ascent to high altitudes.
   - **High-Altitude Pulmonary Edema (HAPE)** and **High-Altitude Cerebral Edema (HACE)** are severe forms of altitude sickness.
   - **Management**: Gradual ascent, acclimatization strategies, descent, supplemental oxygen, and medications (e.g., acetazolamide).

Sports-Specific Injuries

1. **Soccer Injuries**:
   - Commonly involves the lower extremities (e.g., ankle sprains, ACL tears, hamstring strains).
   - Prevention includes proper warm-ups, strength training, and attention to playing surfaces.

2. **Basketball Injuries**:
   - Frequent injuries include ankle sprains, knee injuries (meniscal tears, ACL injuries), and finger dislocations.
   - Focus on plyometric training, balance exercises, and ankle taping for prevention.

3. **Running Injuries**:
   - Overuse injuries like **patellofemoral pain syndrome**, **plantar fasciitis**, **shin splints**, and **stress fractures** are common.
   - Prevention strategies include proper footwear, training modifications, and strength training.

4. **Swimming Injuries**:
   - **Shoulder Injuries (Swimmer's Shoulder)**: Overuse injury due to repetitive overhead movements.
   - **Prevention**: Shoulder strengthening, flexibility training, and proper technique.

5. **Weightlifting Injuries**:
   - Injuries to the lower back, shoulder, and wrist are common due to improper lifting techniques and heavy loads.
   - Emphasizing form, gradual load progression, and core stabilization can help reduce risks.

7. REHABILITATION AND RETURN-TO-PLAY PROTOCOLS

Principles Of Sports Rehabilitation

1. **Individualized Approach**:
    - Every athlete and injury is unique; rehabilitation must be tailored to the athlete's specific needs, sport, and level of competition.
    - Consider the athlete's age, previous injuries, and psychological readiness.

2. **Evidence-Based Practice**:
    - Rehabilitation plans should be based on current best evidence, incorporating techniques that have been proven effective.
    - Regularly update protocols based on emerging research in sports medicine and rehabilitation.

3. **Functional Rehabilitation**:
    - Focus on movements and skills that mimic the athlete's sport to ensure a smooth transition back to play.
    - Address not only the injured tissue but also the kinetic chain, movement patterns, and sport-specific demands.

4. **Multidisciplinary Care**:

- Effective rehabilitation often requires coordination among various professionals, including physicians, physiotherapists, athletic trainers, nutritionists, and mental health specialists.

Phases Of Healing And Rehabilitation Goals

1. **Acute Phase (Inflammatory Phase):**
   - **Duration**: First 48-72 hours after injury.
   - **Goals**:
     - **Control Inflammation**: Use the RICE (Rest, Ice, Compression, Elevation) protocol to minimize swelling and tissue damage.
     - **Pain Management**: NSAIDs may be used as appropriate.
     - **Protect the Injury**: Immobilization or limited weight-bearing may be necessary.

2. **Subacute Phase (Repair and Regeneration Phase):**
   - **Duration**: Lasts from a few days to several weeks.
   - **Goals**:
     - **Promote Healing**: Begin gentle mobilization to improve blood flow and tissue regeneration.
     - **Maintain Range of Motion (ROM)**: Focus on restoring joint flexibility through passive and active ROM exercises.
     - **Introduce Controlled Loading**: Use low-intensity strength exercises to

stimulate tissue healing and prevent atrophy.

3. **Remodeling Phase**:
   - **Duration**: Several weeks to months.
   - **Goals**:
     - **Restore Strength**: Progressively increase strength and resistance exercises.
     - **Improve Function**: Integrate functional movements that resemble sport-specific activities.
     - **Enhance Proprioception and Balance**: Use exercises that target balance, stability, and neuromuscular control to reduce re-injury risk.

4. **Return-to-Activity Phase**:
   - **Goals**:
     - **Achieve Sport-Specific Skills**: Incorporate drills, sprints, jumps, and other relevant movements.
     - **Full Load Tolerance**: Ensure the athlete can safely tolerate the physical demands of the sport without pain or compromised mechanics.

Strength And Conditioning Programs

1. **Progressive Loading**:
   - Gradually increase resistance, repetitions, or duration to build strength while avoiding re-injury.

- Tailor load to the athlete's stage of recovery, sport demands, and individual capacity.

2. **Flexibility and Mobility Training**:
   - Address muscle imbalances and joint restrictions that may contribute to injury.
   - Incorporate dynamic stretching and mobility exercises into rehabilitation sessions.

3. **Aerobic and Anaerobic Conditioning**:
   - Maintain cardiovascular fitness through alternative exercises (e.g., cycling, swimming) that do not stress the injured area.
   - Gradually introduce high-intensity and interval training once appropriate.

4. **Core Stability and Neuromuscular Control**:
   - Core stability exercises enhance overall body control and movement efficiency.
   - Neuromuscular training (e.g., proprioceptive training, balance exercises) can reduce injury recurrence.

Monitoring And Criteria For Return-To-Sport Decisions

1. **Objective Assessment**:
   - Utilize functional tests (e.g., strength tests, balance assessments) and sport-specific movement evaluations.
   - Assess range of motion, joint stability, strength, and neuromuscular control.

2. **Psychological Readiness**:

- Consider the athlete's confidence, fear of re-injury, and mental preparedness to resume full activity.
- Sports psychologists can assist with overcoming psychological barriers.

3. **Load Monitoring**:
- Gradual reintroduction of sport-specific workloads, avoiding sudden spikes that may increase re-injury risk.
- Use wearable technology or manual methods (e.g., training logs) to track workload.

4. **Return-to-Play Criteria**:
- Pain-free movement without compensation.
- Restoration of strength within 90-100% of the uninjured limb or baseline levels.
- Ability to perform sport-specific movements at full speed and intensity.
- Clearance from the medical team after thorough evaluation.

8. PREVENTIVE STRATEGIES IN SPORTS MEDICINE

Warm-Up And Cool-Down Protocols

1. **Warm-Up**:
   - **Purpose**: Prepares the body for physical activity by gradually increasing heart rate, blood flow, muscle temperature, and joint lubrication, reducing the risk of injury.
   - **Components**:
     - **General Warm-Up**: Light aerobic exercises like jogging or cycling to increase body temperature.
     - **Dynamic Stretching**: Incorporate sport-specific movements (e.g., leg swings, arm circles) to activate muscles and improve flexibility and coordination.
   - **Benefits**:
     - Enhances muscle elasticity and range of motion.
     - Prepares muscles and tendons for explosive and high-intensity activity.
     - Improves reaction time and focus for athletes.

2. **Cool-Down**:

- **Purpose**: Facilitates recovery by gradually lowering heart rate and body temperature, reducing muscle soreness, and preventing blood pooling.
- **Components**:
  - **Light Aerobic Activity**: Gentle jogging, walking, or cycling for 5-10 minutes to gradually decrease intensity.
  - **Static Stretching**: Focus on major muscle groups used during activity, holding stretches for 15-30 seconds each.
- **Benefits**:
  - Aids in the removal of metabolic waste (e.g., lactic acid).
  - Reduces muscle stiffness and post-exercise soreness.
  - Promotes relaxation and recovery.

Strength Training, Stretching, And Flexibility Exercises

1. **Strength Training**:
   - **Benefits**:
     - Builds muscular strength, endurance, and power, reducing the risk of muscle strains and tears.
     - Enhances joint stability by strengthening the surrounding musculature.
     - Improves overall athletic performance, including speed,

agility, and balance.

- ◦ **Approach**:
    - ▪ **Periodization**: Cycle strength programs through phases (e.g., hypertrophy, strength, power) to minimize overuse injuries.
    - ▪ **Sport-Specific Exercises**: Focus on exercises that mimic the movements and demands of the athlete's sport.

2. **Stretching and Flexibility**:
    - ◦ **Dynamic Stretching** (Pre-activity):
        - ▪ Enhances flexibility, range of motion, and neuromuscular activation, preparing the body for high-intensity movements.
    - ◦ **Static Stretching** (Post-activity):
        - ▪ Reduces muscle tension and promotes long-term flexibility.
    - ◦ **Proprioceptive Neuromuscular Facilitation (PNF) Stretching**:
        - ▪ A technique combining stretching and muscle contractions to improve flexibility and neuromuscular control.

Nutrition And Hydration For Athletes

1. **Balanced Nutrition**:
    - ◦ **Macronutrients**:
        - ▪ **Carbohydrates**: Primary source of energy during high-intensity sports.

- **Proteins**: Essential for muscle repair, recovery, and growth.
- **Fats**: Important for energy metabolism, especially during endurance activities.
  - **Micronutrients**:
    - Adequate intake of vitamins and minerals, including calcium, vitamin D, iron, and electrolytes, supports bone health, oxygen transport, and metabolic functions.
  - **Meal Timing**:
    - **Pre-Event Nutrition**: High-carbohydrate, moderate-protein meals consumed 3-4 hours before exercise optimize glycogen stores and energy.
    - **Post-Event Recovery**: Emphasize protein and carbohydrate intake within 30 minutes of activity for optimal muscle repair and glycogen replenishment.

2. **Hydration**:
   - **Importance**:
     - Proper hydration maintains body temperature, supports cardiovascular function, and enhances cognitive performance.
   - **Hydration Strategies**:
     - **Pre-Exercise Hydration**: Drink 16-20 ounces of water or a sports drink 2-3 hours before activity.
     - **During Exercise**: Consume fluids

regularly to replace sweat losses.

- **Post-Exercise Rehydration**: Replace fluids lost during exercise, using body weight as a guide for optimal replenishment.

- **Electrolyte Balance**:
  - Replenish sodium, potassium, and other electrolytes lost through sweat to avoid cramping, fatigue, and heat-related conditions.

Sports Psychology And Mental Well-Being

1. **Stress Management**:
   - **Sources of Stress**: Competition pressure, performance anxiety, and balancing sport with life demands can increase stress.
   - **Techniques**:
     - **Mindfulness and Relaxation Exercises**: Breathing techniques, meditation, and progressive muscle relaxation.
     - **Cognitive-Behavioral Strategies**: Techniques for managing negative thoughts and building self-confidence.

2. **Mental Training for Performance**:
   - **Goal Setting**: Establish short-term and long-term goals to maintain motivation and focus.
   - **Visualization and Mental Rehearsal**: Athletes can enhance their skills by mentally practicing scenarios and perfecting

performance techniques.

3. **Psychological Support**:

   - Providing athletes with access to sports psychologists and mental health resources ensures they can handle stress, recover from setbacks, and stay motivated.

   - **Team Dynamics**: Encourage positive team interactions, leadership development, and effective communication.

9. SPECIAL POPULATIONS IN SPORTS MEDICINE

Pediatric And Adolescent Athletes: Growth Plate Injuries And Considerations

1. **Unique Physiology of Young Athletes**:
   - Rapid skeletal growth during adolescence can lead to unique vulnerabilities, including growth plate injuries and muscle imbalances.
   - Hormonal changes influence strength, coordination, and recovery.

2. **Growth Plate (Physeal) Injuries**:
   - **Overview**: Growth plates are areas of developing cartilage near the ends of long bones. They are weaker and more susceptible to injury than surrounding bone, ligaments, or tendons.
   - **Common Injuries**:
     - **Physeal Fractures**: Typically caused by acute trauma (e.g., falls, collisions) and classified using the Salter-Harris classification system.
     - **Overuse Injuries**: Conditions such as **Osgood-Schlatter disease** (tibial tuberosity inflammation) and **Sever's disease** (calcaneal apophysitis) are common due to

repetitive stress.

- ◦ **Management**:
  - ▪ **Prevention**: Encourage rest, proper training techniques, gradual increase in activity intensity, and cross-training to avoid overuse.
  - ▪ **Treatment**: Immobilization, physical therapy, and modified activity levels may be necessary. Surgery is reserved for severe cases.

3. **Considerations for Training**:
   - ◦ Balance strength and flexibility training while avoiding excessive strain on bones and joints.
   - ◦ Emphasize proper technique, adequate nutrition, and rest to support growth and recovery.

Female Athletes: The Female Athlete Triad, Menstrual Health

1. **The Female Athlete Triad**:
   - ◦ **Components**:
     - ▪ **Energy Deficiency with or without Disordered Eating**: Insufficient caloric intake relative to energy expenditure.
     - ▪ **Menstrual Dysfunction**: Ranges from irregular menses to amenorrhea due to hormonal imbalances.
     - ▪ **Bone Health Issues**: Increased risk of low bone mineral density

(osteopenia/osteoporosis), leading to stress fractures.

- ○ **Prevention and Management**:
  - ■ **Multidisciplinary Care**: Involves sports medicine physicians, dietitians, psychologists, and coaches.
  - ■ **Education**: Promote awareness of proper nutrition, caloric balance, and menstrual health.
  - ■ **Monitoring**: Track menstrual cycles and bone health, especially in high-impact sports.

2. **Menstrual Health and Performance**:
   - ○ Menstrual cycle phases can affect physical performance and perceived exertion levels.
   - ○ **Management**: Tailor training loads and rest periods based on menstrual patterns.

Master's Athletes And Aging Population: Managing Age-Related Changes

1. **Physiological Considerations**:
   - ○ **Muscle Mass and Strength Decline**: Sarcopenia (age-related muscle loss) and decreased strength can affect performance and injury risk.
   - ○ **Joint Degeneration**: Increased prevalence of osteoarthritis and other degenerative joint conditions.
   - ○ **Cardiovascular Changes**: Reduced aerobic capacity and slower recovery from high-

intensity efforts.

2. **Training Adaptations**:

   - **Strength and Resistance Training**: Maintains muscle mass, increases bone density, and reduces injury risk.
   - **Recovery Focus**: Allow longer recovery times between training sessions to accommodate slower healing.
   - **Flexibility and Mobility Work**: Incorporate stretching and mobility exercises to maintain range of motion.

3. **Managing Chronic Conditions**:

   - Tailor exercise prescriptions to account for chronic diseases such as hypertension, diabetes, or heart disease.
   - **Injury Prevention**: Use low-impact activities (e.g., swimming, cycling) and gradual progression.

Athletes With Disabilities: Adaptive Sports Medicine

1. **Adaptive Sports**:

   - Inclusive sporting events for athletes with physical, sensory, or intellectual disabilities (e.g., Paralympic Games).
   - **Common Conditions**: May include spinal cord injuries, limb deficiencies, visual impairments, and cerebral palsy.

2. **Injury Patterns and Risk Factors**:

   - Different types of mobility aids, prosthetics, or techniques can contribute to specific overuse injuries or unique biomechanics.

- **Examples**:
  - **Wheelchair Athletes**: Higher incidence of shoulder overuse injuries.
  - **Prosthetic Limb Users**: Potential for skin issues, blisters, and mechanical stress at the interface between residual limb and prosthesis.

3. **Comprehensive Care**:
   - **Multidisciplinary Teams**: Physicians, physical therapists, occupational therapists, orthotists/prosthetists, and psychologists work together to optimize care.
   - **Equipment Modification**: Tailoring devices such as wheelchairs, prosthetics, or orthotics to individual needs can minimize injury risk and enhance performance.
   - **Training Programs**: Focused on strength, endurance, and technical skill development to maximize function and safety.

10. PERFORMANCE ENHANCEMENT AND ETHICAL CONSIDERATIONS

Ergogenic Aids And Doping In Sports

1. **What are Ergogenic Aids?**
   Ergogenic aids are substances or devices used to improve athletic performance. They can be classified into several categories based on their mechanisms of action.

   - **Nutritional Aids**: Vitamins, minerals, amino acids, and protein supplements designed to enhance energy production or recovery.
   - **Mechanical Aids**: Devices like specialized footwear, prosthetics, or equipment designed to improve efficiency and performance.
   - **Pharmacological Aids**: Medications, both legal and illegal, that enhance performance by improving strength, endurance, or recovery.

2. **Doping and Its Impact on Sports**
   Doping refers to the use of banned substances or methods to artificially enhance athletic performance. The **World Anti-Doping Agency (WADA)** oversees the regulation of doping practices and the list of prohibited substances.

- **Common Doping Substances**:
  - **Anabolic Steroids**: Increase muscle mass and strength but have severe side effects, including cardiovascular, hepatic, and psychiatric complications.
  - **Erythropoietin (EPO)**: Enhances red blood cell production to improve endurance, often associated with increased risk of thrombosis.
  - **Human Growth Hormone (HGH)**: Used for muscle repair and regeneration, though its use is banned due to potential long-term health risks.
  - **Stimulants (e.g., amphetamines)**: Used to reduce fatigue and increase alertness but can be addictive and cause cardiovascular issues.

3. **Health Risks of Doping**
   - **Short-Term Risks**: Increased risk of acute cardiovascular events, liver and kidney damage, hormonal imbalances, and psychiatric effects such as aggression or anxiety.
   - **Long-Term Risks**: Chronic health issues such as infertility, cardiovascular disease, and organ damage, along with psychological dependency.
   - **Ethical Concerns**: Doping distorts the fairness of competition, and athletes using banned substances are violating the integrity of sports. Additionally, young athletes who emulate professionals may be

influenced to engage in harmful practices.

4. **Detection and Prevention**

- **Doping Control**: Anti-doping agencies utilize drug testing before, during, and after competition to catch athletes using banned substances.

- **Education and Awareness**: Ensuring athletes and coaches understand the risks and ethical implications of doping is key to prevention.

- **Testing Methods**: Include urine and blood tests, biological passports, and other sophisticated methods to detect performance-enhancing substances.

Supplements And Nutrition

1. **Role of Nutrition in Performance Enhancement**
   Proper nutrition is fundamental to supporting athletic performance, recovery, and long-term health. Well-balanced nutrition enhances endurance, strength, and overall athletic output.

   - **Macronutrients**:

     - **Carbohydrates**: Essential for fueling muscles during endurance sports. Carbohydrate loading before events can improve performance in long-duration activities.

     - **Proteins**: Vital for muscle repair, recovery, and growth. Intake of high-quality protein supports muscle synthesis, particularly post-exercise.

- **Fats**: Provide long-term energy sources, especially in low-intensity sports, and are important for fat-soluble vitamins and hormone production.

- **Micronutrients**:
  - **Vitamins and Minerals**: Essential for metabolic processes and muscle function. For example, vitamin D is crucial for bone health and immune function, while iron supports oxygen delivery to muscles.

2. **Supplements in Sports Medicine**
   While dietary supplements are widely used in sports to improve performance, they should be carefully considered.
   - **Commonly Used Supplements**:
     - **Creatine**: Known to increase muscle strength and power output, particularly in high-intensity, short-duration activities.
     - **Caffeine**: Can enhance endurance by improving focus, reducing fatigue, and increasing fat oxidation.
     - **Branched-Chain Amino Acids (BCAAs)**: Help reduce muscle soreness and support muscle repair after intense workouts.
     - **Beta-Alanine**: Known to buffer lactic acid buildup in muscles, helping improve performance in activities like sprinting or high-intensity interval training.
   - **Risks of Supplements**:

- **Quality Control**: Some supplements are contaminated with banned substances or have impurities that pose health risks.
- **Overuse and Imbalance**: Overreliance on supplements may lead to imbalances in the diet or neglecting the importance of whole foods.
- **Legal Implications**: Some supplements may contain substances banned by WADA, inadvertently resulting in disqualification or suspension for athletes.

3. **Ethical Considerations in Supplementation**
    - **Informed Choice**: Athletes should be fully informed about the supplements they are using, including potential side effects and long-term health consequences.
    - **Equity and Fairness**: The widespread use of certain supplements can lead to an uneven playing field, especially if one athlete has access to more or better-quality supplements than others.

Ethics And Legal Issues In Sports Medicine

1. **Confidentiality and Athlete Privacy**
    - Physicians must maintain confidentiality in all aspects of medical care. This includes medical history, injury details, and any potential use of banned substances.

- Legal considerations include adhering to confidentiality laws (e.g., HIPAA in the U.S.) and obtaining informed consent from athletes when conducting assessments or treatments.

2. **Physician's Role and Conflicts of Interest**

- Sports physicians must prioritize the health and well-being of athletes, sometimes even over performance goals. However, physicians may face pressures from athletes, coaches, or sponsors to provide treatments or guidance that could compromise health for performance enhancement.

- Conflicts of interest must be avoided, and doctors must provide unbiased advice focused on health and recovery, even if it may not align with an athlete's desire to return to play quickly or use potentially harmful performance enhancers.

3. **Legal Issues in Sports Medicine**

- **Malpractice and Liability**: Medical professionals can be held liable for negligence, especially if improper medical advice or failure to report banned substances leads to harm or violates regulations.

- **Doping Regulations**: Athletes and medical professionals must adhere to anti-doping regulations to ensure fairness in competition. Violations can lead to suspensions, fines, and reputational damage.

- **Legal Protections for Athletes**: Some athletes may be unaware of the legal implications of using certain supplements or performance-enhancing drugs, and physicians should educate them to avoid potential legal issues.

4. **The Role of Ethics Committees and Regulatory Bodies**

   ○ Ethical review boards, such as WADA, ethics committees within sports organizations, and professional associations, provide guidelines and oversight to ensure that both athletes and physicians uphold ethical standards in sports medicine.

11. SPECIAL TOPICS IN SPORTS MEDICINE

Sports Medicine In Extreme Sports And Adventure Sports

1. **Overview of Extreme and Adventure Sports**

   Extreme sports and adventure sports are characterized by high levels of physical risk and require athletes to engage in activities that push the limits of their physical and mental endurance. These sports often involve high-speed, high-impact, or altitude-related activities such as rock climbing, mountain biking, snowboarding, surfing, BASE jumping, and skydiving.

2. **Injury Patterns in Extreme Sports**

   - **Trauma and Fractures**: Extreme sports athletes are at a high risk of traumatic injuries such as fractures, dislocations, and head injuries due to the high-impact nature of these activities.

   - **Spinal Injuries**: High-speed sports like skiing, snowboarding, and motocross are associated with a significant risk of cervical and lumbar spine injuries.

   - **Soft Tissue Injuries**: The dynamic movements involved in extreme sports lead to a variety of soft tissue injuries, such as sprains, strains, and contusions, particularly in the upper extremities (e.g., shoulder dislocations in surfing or climbing).

- **Overuse Injuries**: Although less common, extreme sports athletes can also experience overuse injuries, particularly in sports requiring repetitive movements like rock climbing or kayaking.

3. **Risk Mitigation Strategies**

- **Protective Equipment**: Helmets, pads, harnesses, and other protective gear are essential for minimizing injuries. Custom-made equipment can be particularly useful for preventing specific injuries in sports like climbing or BMX racing.

- **Safety Protocols and Training**: Athletes in extreme sports need to undergo specialized safety training to prevent accidents. Coaches and physicians also play a vital role in educating athletes on injury prevention, appropriate warm-ups, and managing fatigue.

- **Emergency Preparedness**: In extreme sports, quick access to medical care is often limited, especially in remote or high-altitude settings. It is crucial for athletes to be trained in basic first aid, and for support staff to have emergency evacuation plans in place.

4. **Rehabilitation and Return to Play in Extreme Sports**
Rehabilitation protocols for extreme sports athletes must be tailored to the sport's unique requirements. The approach should focus not only on physical recovery but also on mental preparedness, as extreme athletes often experience psychological stress after serious injuries. Functional rehabilitation and gradual return-to-play protocols that simulate the conditions of the sport are crucial to ensure the athlete can return

to competition safely.

Role Of Technology: Wearables, Biomechanical Analysis Tools

1. **Wearable Technology in Sports Medicine**
   Wearables have revolutionized the way sports physicians monitor athletes' performance and recovery. These devices provide real-time data on key physiological parameters, allowing for more personalized care.
   - **Types of Wearables**:
     - **Heart Rate Monitors**: Used to assess an athlete's cardiovascular response to training, helping in endurance sports, and ensuring athletes train within optimal heart rate zones.
     - **GPS Trackers**: Common in endurance and team sports, GPS trackers provide insights into athletes' movement patterns, speeds, distances covered, and even workload during training and competition.
     - **Accelerometers**: These devices measure acceleration, providing insight into an athlete's mechanics, force production, and overall physical load, helping to prevent overuse injuries.

2. **Biomechanical Analysis Tools**
   - **Motion Capture Systems**: High-speed cameras and motion sensors are used to capture the movement of athletes, providing

a detailed analysis of their biomechanics. This is crucial for assessing running form, jump mechanics, and the efficiency of movement in various sports.

- **Force Plates**: Force plates measure ground reaction forces during activities such as jumping, running, or landing. They help identify deficiencies in technique that may lead to injury or inefficiency in performance.
- **3D Biomechanical Models**: These advanced systems simulate human movement in three dimensions, offering detailed assessments of joint angles, muscle forces, and postural alignment to help optimize performance and reduce injury risk.

3. **Virtual Reality (VR) and Augmented Reality (AR) in Training**

   VR and AR are increasingly used in sports medicine for both training and rehabilitation. These technologies allow athletes to simulate real-world conditions in a controlled environment, improving their skill development, visual-spatial awareness, and decision-making skills.

4. **Impact on Injury Prevention and Performance Enhancement**

   By providing real-time feedback, wearables and biomechanical analysis tools help identify athletes who may be at risk for injury due to poor mechanics or overtraining. This data can be used to adjust training loads, monitor recovery, and fine-tune performance strategies. This proactive approach can lead to fewer injuries and more efficient training.

E-Sports And Sedentary Injuries

1. **Rise of E-Sports**

   E-sports has become a global phenomenon, with millions of people participating in competitive gaming. Professional gamers can spend long hours sitting and playing, which presents unique challenges for sports medicine professionals. The sedentary nature of gaming, combined with intense focus and rapid hand-eye coordination, can lead to a variety of musculoskeletal, neurological, and psychological issues.

2. **Injuries in E-Sports Athletes**

   While e-sports may not involve traditional physical exertion, the repetitive nature of gameplay can lead to a range of injuries:

   - **Musculoskeletal Injuries:**
     - **Repetitive Strain Injuries (RSI):** E-sports athletes commonly suffer from conditions like **carpal tunnel syndrome**, **tennis elbow**, and **tendinitis** due to long hours of hand and wrist movements.
     - **Postural Issues:** Extended periods of sitting can lead to poor posture, resulting in **neck pain**, **lower back pain**, and **shoulder stiffness**. **Cervical disc herniation** can also occur in severe cases.
   - **Vision Problems: Digital eye strain** and **computer vision syndrome** are common, with symptoms such as dry eyes, headaches, and blurred vision.
   - **Neurological Issues:** Mental fatigue, **stress**, and **sleep disturbances** due to excessive screen time and irregular gaming schedules

can impact cognitive function and overall health.

3. **Preventive Measures in E-Sports**

- **Ergonomics**: Setting up an ergonomic workstation with proper chair support, monitor height, and keyboard positioning can reduce musculoskeletal strain.
- **Scheduled Breaks and Stretching**: Encouraging e-sports athletes to take regular breaks (every 30-60 minutes) to stretch and move can help reduce the risk of injuries.
- **Postural Training**: Teaching proper posture techniques, particularly in the cervical and lumbar spine, can prevent long-term back and neck issues.
- **Mental Health Support**: Addressing mental fatigue and stress through relaxation techniques, proper sleep hygiene, and psychological support can help e-sports athletes maintain their focus and performance.

4. **Role of Sports Medicine in E-Sports**

Sports medicine professionals working with e-sports athletes need to adopt a multidisciplinary approach. This includes addressing physical injuries (musculoskeletal and neurological), mental health issues (stress management, sleep disorders), and the long-term effects of prolonged gaming.

12. 20 CASE STUDIES AND PRACTICAL SCENARIOS

1. Ankle Sprain In A Soccer Player

Case Summary: *A 25-year-old male soccer player presents with pain, swelling, and limited range of motion in his right ankle after an awkward landing during a match.*

He reports hearing a "pop" at the time of injury.

- **Diagnosis**: Ankle sprain (Grade II, lateral ligament complex injury).

- **Management**: Initial R.I.C.E (Rest, Ice, Compression, Elevation), followed by early range-of-motion exercises, physical therapy, and gradual return-to-sport once the athlete is pain-free and demonstrates normal strength and function.

- **Key Takeaways**: Proper assessment of ligamentous injury and the importance of rehabilitation in preventing recurrence.

2. Acl Tear In A Basketball Player

Case Summary: *A 19-year-old female basketball player reports a sudden, severe pain in her knee after a jump and landing on a pivot. She is unable to continue playing and is unable to bear weight on the affected leg.*

- **Diagnosis**: Anterior cruciate ligament (ACL) tear.

- **Management**: MRI to confirm the tear. Surgical intervention (ACL reconstruction) followed by a structured rehabilitation program.

- **Key Takeaways**: Early diagnosis and appropriate surgical management, followed by rehabilitation, are critical for a full recovery and prevention of future knee instability.

3. Tennis Elbow In A Weekend Warrior

Case Summary: *A 35-year-old amateur tennis player complains of pain and tenderness over the lateral epicondyle of the elbow that worsens with gripping activities.*

- **Diagnosis**: Lateral epicondylitis (Tennis Elbow).
- **Management**: Conservative management with rest, ice, anti-inflammatory medications, and physical therapy focusing on eccentric strengthening of the forearm muscles. Corticosteroid injections may be considered if symptoms persist.
- **Key Takeaways**: Tennis elbow is common in recreational athletes, and non-surgical treatment is effective in most cases.

4. Stress Fracture In A Long-Distance Runner

Case Summary: *A 28-year-old female marathon runner presents with gradually increasing pain in her lower leg, especially after running long distances.*

On examination, there is localized tenderness over the tibia.

- **Diagnosis**: Tibial stress fracture.
- **Management**: Rest and modified activity, including a gradual return to running with the use of cross-training modalities such as swimming or cycling. Consideration of bone density testing if the athlete is at risk for osteoporosis.

- **Key Takeaways**: Stress fractures require early diagnosis and appropriate management to avoid complications like non-union or chronic pain.

5. Rotator Cuff Tear In A Baseball Pitcher

Case Summary: *A 30-year-old male baseball pitcher reports shoulder pain, weakness, and difficulty in throwing after a pitch.*
He has had chronic shoulder discomfort that worsened after a recent game.

- **Diagnosis**: Rotator cuff tear (partial thickness).
- **Management**: MRI to confirm the diagnosis. Conservative management with physical therapy focusing on rotator cuff strengthening and scapular stabilization. Surgical intervention may be considered if symptoms persist.
- **Key Takeaways**: Early rehabilitation and activity modification are key to managing rotator cuff injuries. Surgery is reserved for persistent cases.

6. Patellar Tendinopathy In A Volleyball Player

Case Summary: *A 22-year-old female volleyball player presents with pain just below her kneecap, which worsens during jumping and landing.*

- **Diagnosis**: Patellar tendinopathy (Jumper's knee).
- **Management**: Conservative treatment with rest, ice, eccentric strengthening exercises, and patellar tendon loading protocols. If symptoms persist, consider platelet-rich plasma (PRP) injections.
- **Key Takeaways**: Eccentric strengthening is the cornerstone of treatment, and early intervention

prevents chronicity.

7. Achilles Tendon Rupture In A Recreational Sprinter

Case Summary: *A 40-year-old recreational sprinter reports hearing a "pop" and feeling immediate pain in the back of his ankle during a sprint.*

He is unable to push off with his injured leg.

- **Diagnosis**: Achilles tendon rupture.
- **Management**: Diagnosis confirmed with ultrasound or MRI. Surgical or conservative treatment (casting or bracing followed by rehabilitation) depending on the severity and patient preference.
- **Key Takeaways**: Early intervention and appropriate rehabilitation are essential to restoring function after an Achilles tendon rupture.

8. Concussion In A Rugby Player

Case Summary: *A 21-year-old male rugby player loses consciousness briefly after a high tackle.*

He has a headache and nausea but no memory of the incident.

- **Diagnosis**: Concussion (Grade I).
- **Management**: Immediate removal from play and follow the concussion protocol (rest, gradual return-to-play). Cognitive rest, followed by a stepwise return-to-sport protocol once symptom-free.
- **Key Takeaways**: Concussions require careful management and a strict return-to-play protocol to avoid secondary impact syndrome.

9. Plantar Fasciitis In A Crossfit Athlete

Case Summary: *A 30-year-old CrossFit athlete complains of heel pain that is worse in the morning and after prolonged standing.*

- **Diagnosis**: Plantar fasciitis.
- **Management**: Conservative treatment with stretching exercises, orthotics, and night splints. Corticosteroid injections or shockwave therapy may be considered if conservative treatment fails.
- **Key Takeaways**: Early intervention with stretching and footwear modifications can prevent chronic plantar fasciitis.

10. Hamstring Strain In A Football Player

Case Summary: *A 24-year-old male football player experiences sudden pain in his posterior thigh while sprinting during practice.*

- **Diagnosis**: Hamstring strain (Grade II).
- **Management**: Rest, ice, compression, elevation (R.I.C.E.), followed by a progressive rehabilitation program focusing on flexibility and strength.
- **Key Takeaways**: Hamstring strains are common in high-speed sports, and a comprehensive rehabilitation program is key to preventing recurrence.

11. Groin Strain In A Soccer Player

Case Summary: *A 30-year-old male soccer player experiences sharp pain in his groin while attempting a kick during a match.*

- **Diagnosis**: Adductor muscle strain.
- **Management**: R.I.C.E., followed by rehabilitation including stretching and strengthening of the hip

adductors and abdominals.

- **Key Takeaways**: Groin strains require careful rehabilitation to restore strength and flexibility while avoiding further injury.

12. Meniscal Tear In A Skiing Accident

Case Summary: *A 45-year-old male skier falls and twists his knee during a downhill run, reporting pain, swelling, and difficulty bending the knee.*

- **Diagnosis**: Medial meniscal tear.
- **Management**: MRI for confirmation, followed by conservative management (rest, ice, bracing) or surgical intervention (meniscectomy or repair) depending on the severity and symptoms.
- **Key Takeaways**: Meniscal tears can be managed conservatively in some cases, but surgery may be necessary for persistent or complex tears.

13. Low Back Pain In A Weightlifter

Case Summary: *A 28-year-old male weightlifter presents with acute lower back pain after performing a deadlift.*
He has difficulty standing upright and experiences pain with movement.

- **Diagnosis**: Lumbar strain.
- **Management**: Rest, ice, and anti-inflammatory medication followed by physical therapy. Gradual return to training with proper lifting techniques and core strengthening exercises.
- **Key Takeaways**: Proper lifting techniques and core stability exercises are crucial in preventing low back injuries in weightlifters.

14. Hip Labral Tear In A Dancer

Case Summary: *A 19-year-old female ballet dancer complains of groin pain and stiffness after an intense rehearsal.*

- **Diagnosis**: Hip labral tear.
- **Management**: MRI for confirmation. Conservative treatment with physical therapy focused on strengthening the hip muscles. Surgical intervention may be necessary for significant tears.
- **Key Takeaways**: Early diagnosis and rehabilitation are key to managing hip labral tears, especially in athletes involved in repetitive motion sports like dance.

15. It Band Syndrome In A Marathon Runner

Case Summary: *A 40-year-old male marathon runner presents with lateral knee pain that worsens after running long distances.*

- **Diagnosis**: Iliotibial band (ITB) syndrome.
- **Management**: Conservative treatment with stretching of the IT band, strengthening of hip abductors, and modification of running mechanics.
- **Key Takeaways**: ITB syndrome is common in runners and can be prevented with proper stretching and strength training.

16. Scoliosis In A Teenage Athlete

Case Summary: *A 15-year-old female gymnast is diagnosed with scoliosis during a routine sports physical examination.*
She reports occasional back pain but no other symptoms.

- **Diagnosis**: Adolescent idiopathic scoliosis.

- **Management**: Monitoring and regular follow-up, with the consideration of bracing if the curve worsens. Avoidance of high-impact activities that exacerbate spinal curvature.
- **Key Takeaways**: Scoliosis in athletes requires careful monitoring to prevent long-term complications, but many athletes can continue to participate in sports with appropriate management.

17. Shin Splints In A Track Athlete

Case Summary: *A 20-year-old male track athlete reports pain along the shin during and after running, particularly during intense sprinting sessions.*

- **Diagnosis**: Medial tibial stress syndrome (Shin splints).
- **Management**: Rest, ice, and correction of running form. Gradual return to running with attention to footwear and training loads.
- **Key Takeaways**: Shin splints are common in runners, and early intervention with load management is crucial to avoid progression to stress fractures.

18. Shoulder Impingement Syndrome In A Swimmer

Case Summary: *A 22-year-old male competitive swimmer presents with shoulder pain and weakness, particularly with overhead movements.*

- **Diagnosis**: Shoulder impingement syndrome.
- **Management**: Conservative treatment with physical

therapy focusing on strengthening the rotator cuff and scapular stabilizers. Avoidance of overhead activities until recovery.

- **Key Takeaways**: Early rehabilitation and correction of swimming technique are crucial in managing shoulder impingement.

19. Dislocated Shoulder In A Rugby Player

Case Summary: *A 27-year-old male rugby player sustains a shoulder dislocation after a tackle.*

- **Diagnosis**: Anterior shoulder dislocation.
- **Management**: Reduction of the dislocation followed by rehabilitation focusing on shoulder stability and prevention of recurrence.
- **Key Takeaways**: Shoulder dislocations require prompt reduction and rehabilitation to restore function and prevent recurrent injuries.

20. Overtraining Syndrome In A Competitive Cyclist

Case Summary: *A 35-year-old competitive cyclist presents with fatigue, poor performance, and irritability after several months of intense training.*

- **Diagnosis**: Overtraining syndrome.
- **Management**: Rest and recovery, with a gradual return to training. Psychological support may also be needed to address the mental and emotional aspects of overtraining.
- **Key Takeaways**: Overtraining syndrome requires a multifaceted approach involving rest, psychological support, and a balanced training regimen.

13.DIAGNOSTIC CHALLENGES AND COMPLEX CASES IN SPORTS MEDICINE

1. Scenario: Chronic Ankle Pain In A Competitive Runner

Case Overview:

A 28-year-old competitive marathon runner presents with a history of chronic right ankle pain, persisting for several months.

The pain is localized around the lateral malleolus and is aggravated by running, especially during long distances. Despite rest and physical therapy, the pain has not improved.

There is no obvious swelling or bruising, and the runner has a normal gait during the physical exam.

The patient has been diagnosed previously with a sprained ankle, but symptoms continue to persist.

Diagnostic Challenge:

The patient's symptoms suggest chronic lateral ankle instability or possibly tendinopathy. However, the persistent nature of the pain despite conservative treatment raises suspicion for a more complex issue.

Key Points in Diagnosis:

- **Clinical History**: The athlete's detailed training history and the onset of symptoms after a specific incident (e.g., an acute sprain during a race) could suggest post-traumatic arthritis or cartilage damage. It's also important to understand the type and intensity of the running regimen, as overuse injuries like tendinopathies are common in long-distance runners.

- **Physical Exam**: While the lack of swelling and bruising may suggest no recent trauma, signs of instability such as anterior or posterior drawer tests for the ankle should be performed to rule out ligamentous injury.

- **Imaging and Testing**:
  - **X-rays** to rule out fractures or signs of early arthritis.
  - **MRI** is more definitive, as it can show soft tissue damage such as ligament tears, tendon inflammation, or early cartilage changes that might not be visible on X-ray.
  - **Ultrasound**: Useful in evaluating tendon injuries, particularly to detect tendinopathies or tears in the peroneal tendons, which could explain the lateral ankle pain.

Diagnosis and Management:

- **Diagnosis**: MRI reveals mild degenerative changes in the talonavicular joint (early arthritis) and mild peroneal tendinopathy. The combination of mechanical and overuse factors has contributed to the chronic nature of the injury.

- **Management**: A multifaceted treatment plan is required, including:
  - Rest and a period of reduced mileage.
  - Use of orthotics to stabilize the foot and prevent excessive stress on the lateral ankle.
  - Physical therapy focusing on strengthening and proprioception exercises to address underlying instability.
  - If conservative treatment fails, surgical options such as tendon debridement or joint

arthroscopy may be considered.

2. Scenario: Shoulder Pain In A College Baseball Player

Case Overview:

A 21-year-old collegiate baseball player reports pain in his throwing shoulder.

The pain started after an increase in the intensity of his training program, particularly focusing on long-toss and throwing at higher velocities.

The athlete experiences discomfort with overhead movements and pain when reaching behind his back.

There is mild weakness, but no numbness or tingling.

The physical exam reveals pain with shoulder flexion, abduction, and external rotation, but no visible deformity or instability.

Diagnostic Challenge:

Shoulder pain in overhead athletes like baseball players can result from a variety of conditions, including rotator cuff injuries, labral tears, and impingement syndrome. The absence of significant weakness or sensory changes complicates the diagnosis, as these symptoms may not clearly point to one condition over another.

Key Points in Diagnosis:

- **Clinical History**: The increase in training intensity and the specific mechanism of injury (overhead throwing) raises suspicion for rotator cuff strain or impingement. Additionally, it's important to assess whether the athlete has a history of any shoulder instability or previous dislocations, which may predispose to labral tears.

- **Physical Exam:**
    - **Neer's and Hawkins-Kennedy Tests** are used to assess for shoulder impingement.

- Apprehension Test is used to evaluate for glenohumeral instability.
- Drop Arm Test to evaluate the function of the rotator cuff muscles.

- Imaging and Testing:
  - X-rays to rule out fractures, dislocations, or any bony changes indicative of impingement.
  - MRI with contrast (arthrogram) to assess for labral tears, rotator cuff injuries, or other soft tissue damage.
  - Ultrasound can be used for dynamic assessment of rotator cuff pathology or impingement.

Diagnosis and Management:

- Diagnosis: MRI reveals a small partial-thickness tear of the supraspinatus tendon (rotator cuff tear) and mild anterior labral fraying. The player likely has a combination of impingement and rotator cuff tendinopathy.

- Management:
  - Conservative Approach: A trial of rest, anti-inflammatory medications, and physical therapy focusing on rotator cuff strengthening and scapular stabilization exercises.
  - Surgical Options: If symptoms persist after conservative management, arthroscopic surgery may be considered to address the rotator cuff tear and any labral pathology.

3. Scenario: Unexplained Leg Pain In A High School

Basketball Player

Case Overview:

A 17-year-old high school basketball player presents with gradual onset of diffuse pain in the lower leg, particularly in the tibial region.

The pain is worse with activity and improves with rest. The athlete denies any recent trauma but reports frequent jumping and running during practice sessions.

There is tenderness over the medial tibial border, but no obvious swelling or deformity.

The patient has been given a diagnosis of shin splints but has not responded to typical treatment.

Diagnostic Challenge:

While the diagnosis of shin splints (medial tibial stress syndrome) is common in athletes involved in running sports, persistent symptoms despite rest and treatment could indicate another underlying condition, such as stress fractures or compartment syndrome.

Key Points in Diagnosis:

- **Clinical History**: The athlete's participation in high-intensity jumping sports such as basketball, combined with the gradual onset of pain, suggests overuse injury, but the persistence of symptoms raises suspicion for other conditions.

- **Physical Exam**:
  - Tenderness localized to the tibial shaft could indicate stress fractures, especially when point tenderness is noted.
  - The absence of swelling and the vague nature of the pain could also point to compartment syndrome, though it typically presents with more intense pain and potential nerve involvement.

- **Imaging and Testing**:
  - **X-rays** may miss early stress fractures, so further imaging like a **bone scan** or **MRI** may be necessary to detect microfractures.
  - **MRI** can reveal stress fractures in the tibia, stress reactions, and potential signs of compartment syndrome.

Diagnosis and Management:

- **Diagnosis**: MRI reveals a stress fracture in the medial tibial shaft, likely exacerbated by repetitive stress from basketball training.
- **Management**:
  - **Conservative Treatment**: Rest and activity modification, including cross-training with non-weight-bearing exercises (e.g., swimming or cycling).
  - **Casting** or use of a walking boot may be required for immobilization.
  - Gradual return to sport with a structured rehabilitation program focusing on strengthening and biomechanical correction to prevent recurrence.

4. Scenario: Compartment Syndrome In An Ultra-Endurance Athlete

Case Overview:

A 32-year-old ultra-endurance athlete presents with severe leg pain and swelling after completing a 100-mile race.

The athlete has been running for several years and has not experienced such pain before.

The pain is most pronounced in the anterior compartment of the lower leg, with a feeling of tightness and an inability to continue running.

The pain worsens with activity and is not relieved by rest. The athlete also reports numbness and tingling in the foot.

Diagnostic Challenge:

This case presents a typical scenario for acute compartment syndrome, but the diagnosis can be difficult due to the potential overlap with other conditions, such as muscle strain or rhabdomyolysis. Additionally, compartment syndrome can be challenging to diagnose in the absence of clear signs of external trauma.

Key Points in Diagnosis:

- **Clinical History**: The recent intense activity (ultra-endurance race) and the combination of tightness, swelling, and nerve-related symptoms (numbness and tingling) are key clues pointing toward compartment syndrome.

- **Physical Exam:**
    - **Palpation** may reveal tight, firm compartments, especially in the anterior tibial area.
    - **Pain out of proportion** to the injury and increased pain with passive stretching of the affected muscles.

- **Imaging and Testing:**
    - **Intra-compartmental pressure measurement** is the gold standard for diagnosing compartment syndrome. Pressures >30-40 mmHg are indicative of the condition.
    - **MRI** can be used to evaluate the extent of muscle swelling, though it is not diagnostic for compartment syndrome itself.

Diagnosis and Management:

- **Diagnosis:**   Intra-compartmental   pressure measurements confirm acute compartment syndrome.

- **Management**:
    - ◦ **Surgical Intervention**: Immediate fasciotomy is necessary to relieve pressure and prevent permanent muscle and nerve damage.
    - ◦ **Post-Surgical Care**: Monitoring for complications such as infection, muscle necrosis, and nerve damage, with rehabilitation focused on restoring function.

14.ETHICAL DILEMMAS IN SPORTS MEDICINE: REAL-WORLD SCENARIOS

1. Scenario: Return To Play After Concussion

Case Overview:
A 23-year-old professional football player sustains a concussion during a game after a hard tackle.

He briefly loses consciousness but returns to the game after passing a sideline concussion assessment.

Over the next few days, he reports persistent mild headaches, difficulty concentrating, and occasional dizziness.

However, he insists that he feels "fine" and is eager to return to play, as the team is in a critical position for playoffs.

His coach and team doctors are under pressure to clear him for the upcoming match.

Ethical Dilemma:
The ethical challenge is whether the athlete should be cleared to return to play when there are lingering concussion symptoms. There is pressure from both the athlete and the team to return quickly, but returning too soon could increase the risk of second-impact syndrome or long-term neurological damage.

Key Considerations:

- **Athlete's Autonomy vs. Medical Advice**: The athlete's desire to play might conflict with medical advice to rest and recover. It's essential to balance the athlete's wishes with the medical team's responsibility to protect the athlete from further harm.

- **Informed Consent**: The athlete should be fully informed of the risks of returning to play too soon, including potential long-term cognitive effects, and be involved in the decision-making process.
- **Best Interest of the Athlete**: The primary concern must be the athlete's health, not team performance or pressure to return to competition.

Management and Resolution:

- The medical team, following the latest concussion management protocols (e.g., graduated return-to-play process), must decide not to clear the athlete for play until they have fully recovered. Despite the athlete's and team's desires to return him to competition, the decision is based on the principle of "do no harm" to ensure his long-term neurological health.
- Ethical guidelines and the importance of player safety must take precedence over performance goals. The medical team must communicate openly with the athlete, providing a clear rationale for the decision.

2. Scenario: Balancing Player Safety With Team Performance

Case Overview:

A 30-year-old professional soccer player has been playing with a chronic knee injury (mild ACL tear) that has not required surgery but causes discomfort during play.

The injury has been managed conservatively with physiotherapy and occasional injections.

The player has a pivotal role on the team, and with an important match approaching, the coach and team management are pressuring the medical staff to clear him to play despite his ongoing pain.

Ethical Dilemma:

The dilemma here is whether to prioritize the team's immediate performance over the player's long-term well-being. The athlete is at risk of further damage to the knee, which could lead to a more serious injury that may require surgical intervention and a prolonged recovery period.

Key Considerations:

- **Duty of Care**: The medical team has a duty to protect the athlete's long-term health, even when it may negatively impact team performance. This means considering the potential for worsening the injury and the risk of disabling the athlete long-term.
- **Informed Decision-Making**: The athlete needs to be fully informed of the potential consequences of continuing to play with the knee injury, including the risk of permanent damage, and given the opportunity to make an informed decision about his own health.
- **Team Pressure**: Team performance objectives, such as winning a championship, may conflict with the need for proper injury management. This introduces the risk that performance pressures could unduly influence medical decisions.

Management and Resolution:

- The medical team should conduct a thorough evaluation, including imaging studies (e.g., MRI) to assess the extent of the injury. If the risk of further damage is deemed significant, the player should not be cleared to play.
- A clear communication strategy should be used to explain to the athlete, coach, and management that player safety is paramount and that a full recovery is in

the best interest of both the player and the team in the long run.

- In cases like this, the physician's primary ethical responsibility is to protect the athlete from harm, even if it means disappointing the team.

3. Scenario: Athlete's Autonomy Vs. Medical Advice In Treatment Choices

Case Overview:
A 26-year-old female tennis player presents with chronic shoulder pain that has been interfering with her performance.

After a series of imaging tests, the diagnosis is a labral tear, and the medical team recommends surgery to correct the issue.

However, the player is adamant that she does not want surgery and prefers to manage the condition with conservative treatments, such as cortisone injections and physical therapy.

Her coach and team managers are supportive of this decision, as they want her to return to competitive play as soon as possible.

Ethical Dilemma:
In this case, the dilemma is between respecting the athlete's autonomy and medical advice. The player wants to avoid surgery due to the risks and recovery time involved, but the medical team knows that her decision may lead to prolonged pain and long-term damage to the shoulder, potentially ending her career early.

Key Considerations:
- **Respect for Autonomy**: The player has the right to make decisions about her own body, even if those decisions may not align with the physician's recommendation. It is crucial that the player is fully informed about the potential risks and benefits of the

options, including conservative management versus surgery.

- **Best Interest of the Athlete**: The medical team must consider whether the player's decision is in her best long-term interests. This includes explaining the potential consequences of delaying or avoiding surgery.
- **Pressure from Coaches and Managers**: There may be external pressures to return to play as soon as possible, which can cloud the decision-making process. The medical team must ensure that the decision is driven by the athlete's well-being, not by team performance or external pressure.

Management and Resolution:

- The physician should engage in a thorough discussion with the player, explaining the potential risks of continued conservative management, including the possibility of worsening the tear or developing additional injuries.
- A second opinion or referral to a specialist could also be offered to ensure the athlete is well-informed.
- Ultimately, the decision should be made based on the athlete's informed consent, but with ongoing support and monitoring from the medical team to ensure that any progression of the injury is addressed early on.

4. Scenario: Managing Doping Concerns In A Young Athlete

Case Overview:
A 19-year-old sprinter is caught using a banned substance during routine drug testing at a track and field competition.

The athlete insists that they did not knowingly take the drug, claiming it was in a supplement they bought online.

The athlete is a rising star, with the potential to qualify for the national team, and there is substantial pressure from sponsors, coaches, and fans to protect the athlete's career.

The medical staff is aware that the athlete's use of performance-enhancing substances could have serious long-term health implications.

Ethical Dilemma:
The ethical dilemma here centers on the responsibility of the medical team to uphold ethical standards and prevent harm while balancing the athlete's career aspirations and external pressures. Should the medical team advocate for the athlete's future success, potentially overlooking the substance violation, or should they enforce strict adherence to anti-doping rules, which could jeopardize the athlete's career?

Key Considerations:

- **Duty to Uphold Integrity and Health**: The medical team has an ethical obligation to uphold the integrity of the sport and protect the athlete's health by adhering to anti-doping regulations.

- **Consequences of Doping**: The long-term health risks of performance-enhancing drugs must be communicated, including hormonal imbalances, organ damage, and potential for addiction. The short-term career benefits do not outweigh the risks to the athlete's long-term well-being.

- **Athlete's Autonomy and Career**: While the athlete has the right to make decisions about their own career, the medical staff must act as advocates for their long-term health and safety, ensuring that they fully understand the consequences of their actions.

Management and Resolution:

- The medical team must follow ethical guidelines and regulatory standards regarding doping, ensuring that the athlete is held accountable for the use of banned substances.
- Education about the dangers of performance-enhancing drugs and the importance of clean sport should be part of the conversation, and the athlete should be offered support in understanding how to reach their goals safely.
- Depending on the level of violation and the athlete's explanation, a formal sanction may be necessary, but the medical team should provide counseling and guidance to help the athlete avoid similar issues in the future.

15. FUTURE TRENDS AND INNOVATIONS IN SPORTS MEDICINE

1. Emerging Treatments And Regenerative Medicine

Stem Cells in Sports Medicine

Stem cell therapy has gained attention in the treatment of musculoskeletal injuries, particularly in cases where traditional treatments have been unsuccessful.

The potential for stem cells to regenerate damaged tissues offers new hope for athletes with chronic conditions or severe injuries, such as tendonitis, cartilage degeneration, and ligament tears.

- **Mechanism**: Stem cells have the ability to differentiate into different types of cells, including cartilage, bone, and muscle cells. By injecting stem cells into injured areas, the hope is that these cells will promote healing and tissue regeneration.

- **Applications**: Stem cell therapy is being used in the treatment of tendon injuries (e.g., Achilles tendonitis), joint degeneration (e.g., osteoarthritis), and cartilage repair. Early studies suggest positive results, though further research is needed to validate the long-term efficacy.

- **Challenges and Considerations**: One of the main concerns with stem cell therapy is the lack of standardized protocols, inconsistent outcomes, and potential for complications. The regulatory landscape for stem cell therapies is still developing, and ethical issues, such as sourcing of stem cells, remain important considerations.

Platelet-Rich Plasma (Prp) Therapy

PRP therapy involves using a patient's own blood to concentrate platelets and growth factors that promote healing.

It has gained popularity as a treatment for a variety of musculoskeletal injuries, particularly tendinopathies, ligament sprains, and cartilage degeneration.

- **Mechanism**: Blood is drawn from the patient, processed to concentrate platelets, and then injected into the injured area. The high concentration of growth factors in PRP is believed to enhance tissue healing.

- **Applications**: PRP is commonly used for tendon injuries (e.g., tennis elbow, rotator cuff injuries), ligament sprains, and osteoarthritis. It is also explored for muscle injuries and chronic conditions that do not respond well to conservative treatments.

- **Challenges and Considerations**: While PRP has shown promise in clinical trials, the evidence is still mixed on its effectiveness for some conditions. Standardizing the preparation and injection protocols remains an ongoing issue. Additionally, PRP is considered a relatively expensive treatment, which could limit its accessibility.

2. Advances In Surgical Techniques And Robotics

Minimally Invasive Surgery (Mis)

Minimally invasive surgery involves making smaller incisions, which leads to less trauma to the tissues, reduced pain, and faster recovery times compared to traditional open surgeries.

In sports medicine, MIS techniques have revolutionized the management of joint, tendon, and ligament injuries.

- **Applications**: MIS is commonly used in procedures like arthroscopy (for knee, shoulder, and hip surgeries), ligament repairs, and rotator cuff surgeries. The smaller incisions reduce scarring, risk of infection, and recovery time, allowing athletes to return to competition more quickly.

- **Advantages**: The benefits of MIS include decreased pain, reduced blood loss, and shorter hospital stays. It also promotes quicker rehabilitation, which is crucial for athletes aiming for a fast return to their sport.

- **Challenges and Considerations**: While MIS provides many benefits, it requires a high level of surgical skill and specialized equipment. There may be limitations in dealing with more complex injuries, requiring a balance between minimally invasive and traditional approaches.

Robotic-Assisted Surgery

Robotic-assisted surgery in sports medicine is an exciting frontier, providing surgeons with enhanced precision, control, and visualization during procedures. Robotics are particularly useful in joint replacement surgeries, tendon repairs, and arthroscopic procedures.

- **Applications**: Robotic surgery has been most widely applied in knee and hip replacement surgeries, but its use is expanding to more complex procedures such as ligament reconstructions and meniscal repairs. Robots can offer better precision in bone alignment, which is essential in joint replacement surgeries.

- **Advantages**: Robotic systems allow for highly precise cuts, minimizing damage to surrounding tissues and improving post-operative recovery. Enhanced visualization and real-time imaging capabilities enable surgeons to make more accurate decisions during surgery.
- **Challenges and Considerations**: The cost of robotic systems is high, which may limit access to these technologies in some settings. Training and expertise are also necessary for effective use, and there is ongoing research to fully understand the long-term benefits and potential complications associated with robotic surgery.

3. Ai And Data Analytics In Sports Performance And Injury Prevention

Artificial Intelligence (Ai) In Sports Medicine

AI technologies are increasingly being utilized to analyze sports performance, predict injuries, and enhance training regimens.

Machine learning algorithms can process vast amounts of data to identify patterns that might not be apparent to the human eye, enabling more personalized and proactive care.

- **Applications**: AI can be used to analyze biomechanics during training and competition, detect early signs of overtraining, and predict the risk of injury. For example, AI can assess an athlete's gait, running form, or movement patterns and flag any irregularities that could lead to an injury.

- **Predictive Injury Modeling**: AI-based systems are now being developed to predict injury risks by analyzing factors like training load, fatigue levels, biomechanics, and even psychological state. These systems can provide valuable insights into an athlete's readiness to compete and prevent injuries by adjusting their training program.

- **Performance Optimization**: AI can also be used to optimize performance by analyzing data from various sensors (e.g., heart rate, movement trackers, muscle fatigue) to adjust training intensity and recovery times based on the athlete's condition.

Data Analytics In Injury Prevention

Data analytics in sports medicine involves the collection and analysis of data from wearable devices, motion sensors, and biomechanics tools to monitor an athlete's physical condition in real-time.

This allows for more informed decisions regarding training intensity, workload, and recovery strategies.

- **Applications**: Wearable technology, such as GPS trackers and accelerometers, can track the athlete's movements, heart rate, and workload during training. This data is then analyzed to detect early signs of fatigue or improper movement patterns that could lead to injury.

- **Real-Time Feedback**: Coaches and sports medical professionals can use data analytics to adjust training plans in real-time, reducing the risk of overtraining or improper technique. For example, if an athlete's motion patterns indicate increased risk for an ACL tear, their training can be modified to address this issue before an injury occurs.

Challenges And Considerations:

- **Data Security and Privacy**: With the rise in wearable technology and data collection, ensuring the privacy and security of athletes' personal data is crucial. Strict protocols and regulations will be required to safeguard sensitive information.
- **Interpretation of Data**: While AI and data analytics offer immense potential, interpreting the data accurately remains a challenge. Ensuring that athletes and medical professionals understand the insights generated by AI systems is key to making effective, evidence-based decisions.

Ethical And Legal Considerations

With the rapid advancements in sports medicine, ethical and legal concerns are becoming more pronounced.

These include questions about the long-term safety of emerging treatments like stem cell therapy and PRP, the role of AI in making medical decisions, and the balance between enhancing performance and maintaining fairness in sports.

- **Regulation of New Treatments**: Emerging therapies such as stem cell treatments and gene therapy require careful regulation to ensure patient safety and efficacy. Unproven treatments that promise rapid recovery must be scrutinized to avoid harm to athletes.
- **Fairness and Doping**: The use of regenerative therapies to speed up recovery raises questions about whether it gives athletes an unfair advantage. As treatments become more advanced, it may become harder to distinguish between legitimate recovery and

performance enhancement.

- **AI in Decision-Making**: As AI plays a larger role in diagnosing and managing injuries, questions about accountability, reliability, and bias in AI models will need to be addressed to ensure ethical use in sports medicine.

ABOUT THE AUTHOR

Dr Essam Abdelhakim

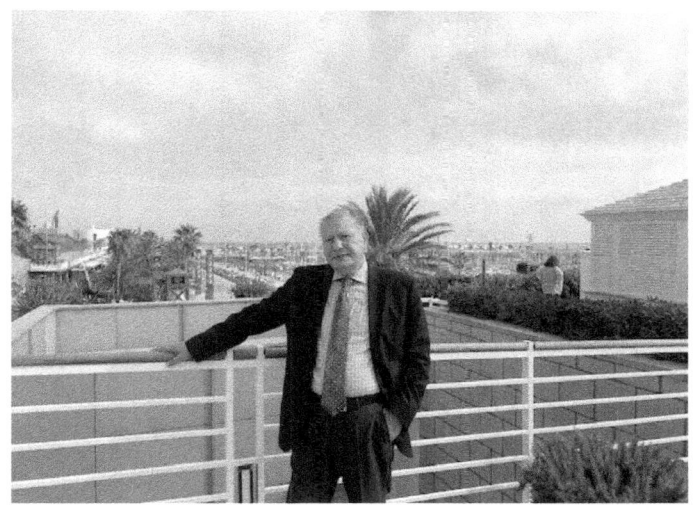

Senior Consultant and Expert in Medical Education

DISCLOSURE

Disclosure

This book has been created with the assistance of *Artificial Intelligence (AI) tools* and thoroughly reviewed and edited by the author to ensure clarity, relevance, and educational value.

While every effort has been made to provide accurate and up-to-date information, this content is intended solely for educational and informational purposes.

The author is a medical professional; however, the information provided in this book *is not a substitute for professional medical advice, diagnosis, or treatment.*

Readers are strongly advised to consult licensed healthcare providers or specialists for any medical concerns or conditions.

By using this book, **you acknowledge and agree** that the author shall not be held responsible or liable for any loss, damage, or harm whether physical, emotional, financial, or otherwise that may occur *as a result of the use or misuse of the information presented herein.*

www.ingramcontent.com/pod-product-compliance
Lightning Source LLC
Chambersburg PA
CBHW070111230526
45472CB00004B/1222